I'LL WALK TOMORROW

By

Roger Winter

The Warner Press
Anderson, Indiana

Dedicated with affection
to my wife, Tres,
to our daughter, Lori,
to relatives and friends,
who in their ways make my life
a happy one!

Contents

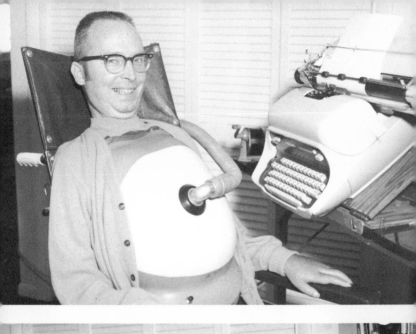

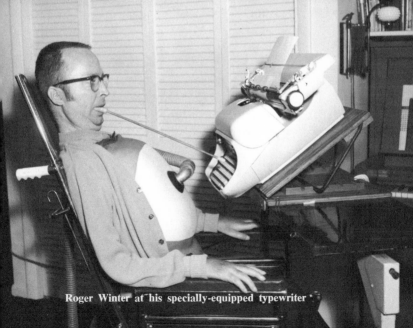

Roger Winter at his specially-equipped typewriter

Chapter *1*

Like It Was

The morning I awoke in the hospital, completely paralyzed and in an iron lung, I didn't know where I was or what day it was. My conscious mind kept saying "Unreal! Unreal!" but my senses revealed its reality. There was the unmistakably antiseptic hospital smell, the rythmic sound of the lung pumping, and the dry-mouth taste as the result of a fever. It was a little like waking in the middle of a bad dream to find that the dream was actually real.

This was the beginning of a pivot-point in my life. It was in August of 1952, that I walked into Memorial Hospital with what the doctor diagnosed as polio. I had just turned twenty-one and was eagerly anticipating my senior year at Kalamazoo College (Kalamazoo, Michigan). In fact, it was only a week prior to reporting for football practice that I developed what I thought was just a heavy cold. Little did I foresee the change that was about to take place in my life, a change in all areas.

The results of that change are the reason I have undertaken the effort of a second book. My first, *Point After Touchdown,* described in detail the sequence of events from my childhood to some twelve years after polio. The first chapter of this book is a brief look at those events. To better disclose the vantage point from which I am writing, I feel it necessary to tell it like it *was* before I tell it like it *is!* It all began right here in South Bend, Indiana.

PRETEEN-AGE YEARS

Born in June of 1931, I moved with my family to Los Angeles, California, when I was six months old. A year-and-a-half later, following one of California's more severe earthquakes, we returned to South Bend, where I grew up.

The early years were typical of most boys during that era. It was full of Cowboys and Indians, cops and robbers, "ducks on the pond," and "tap the icebox." There was the fascination with radio heroes: Jack Armstrong, Captain Midnight, the Lone Ranger, plus secret codes, box tops, and special gadget toys. Climbing trees, making rubber-guns from old inner tubes, building scooters out of orange crates and roller skate wheels—these were just a few of our favorite activities. There were always plenty of neighborhood friends around on East Fairview Street to pursue most any whim that came to mind, ranging from pranks to good deeds.

My grandfather and cousin lived with us during these years. With five of us at home there was always something going on. I would often accompany my dad and grandfather on a hunting excursion on a brisk fall Saturday afternoon through woods ablaze with color. Or, we might take a day to go fishing over on Hudson Lake just west of town. Every summer we rented a cottage at one of the nearby lakes for two weeks— except for the couple of summers I attended the YMCA Camp Eberhart. The holidays brought large gatherings and many presents. Family reunions, held each year near Bremen, Indiana, brought some forty to fifty of my relatives together.

There also were chores typical of the times. Carrying the ashes up from the basement was one of those "I-hate-it" jobs. Cleaning the basement floor after several tons of coal had been dumped into the coal bin, was not something I looked forward to either. My grandfather, a farmer all his life, took to raising rabbits in the garage. When I was old enough, watering and feeding the rabbits became a way I earned a little spending money. One time, pigs were added to our "garage-barn," but neighbors finally put a halt to the farm granddad was creating in the city.

Entering school in 1936 brought me mixed emotions. The first day in kindergarten at James Monroe School was traumatic. I did not want to go and fought, cried, and tried to get out of staying. The days, months, and years in school that followed were difficult. Certainly nothing more than an average student, I was almost retained a year in the fourth grade. Because of shyness I disliked reciting in class and was afraid to ask questions of the teachers. With embarrassment, I recall yet the day I desperately needed to go to the rest room but was afraid to ask permission. The janitor soon had to bring a mop to dry the floor under my desk!

Toward the end of the elementary years, I discovered an interest in which to excel. Clifford Barnes, then gym instructor and basketball coach at Monroe, encouraged me to join the tumbling team. In the sixth grade I tried out for the basketball team and made it. Though small in stature, I soon learned that quickness and speed were assets in any sport. I began to gain confidence in myself, having learned that I could attain praise and recognition. When I became captain of the City Basketball Champions in the seventh grade, my ego received a real boost.

During this same time, however, problems developed at home. My parents divorced. My mother remarried, and I continued to live with my father and cousin. As a twelve-year-old who'd had a rather happy childhood, I found this experience most unsettling. At the time, I did not understand such complicated adult relationships, so the future seemed very uncertain. I also soon left James Monroe Elementary School and entered the rapidly-paced years of secondary school.

HIGH SCHOOL TO COLLEGE

Walking the hallowed halls of Riley High School the first day as an eighth grader, I was somewhat overwhelmed. My active interest in sports had acquainted me with the names of many football and basketball stars. To think that I would be brushing shoulders and practicing on the same field with such heroes was almost beyond my wildest imagination. A whole new world began to unfold.

Neighborhood friends gradually were replaced by new acquaintances at school, especially those interested in sports. Homelife also was changing. My father purchased a tavern, making it necessary for him and my cousin to work afternoons and evenings. Because there was no family at home to go to each day after school, I began to seek the security of friends. There had been no association with church except on an occasional basis. God, to me, was a remote image of a Santa Claus of whom one might ask a favor. I prayed from time to time for such things as winning a ball game, dating a certain girl, obtaining a good test grade. Religion ran a poor last in life for me. I saw no need or reason to have faith in God.

In my freshman year at Riley, things began to happen. I was elected president of the class (because my name was easier to spell than the classmate I ran against), and launched out into football where we won the City Junior High Championship.

13

The following year I had one of my most thrilling experiences in sports. Spike Kelly, head football coach, allowed several of us sophomores playing on the B Team to dress for a varsity game. Near the end of the game, when we had a substantial lead, Spike sent me in with a play.

It was a run around right end and I was to carry the ball. I actually trembled as the huddle broke, we lined up, and the quarterback began barking signals. Before I had time to fully comprehend what was actually happening, the ball was snapped into my hands and several blockers began clearing a path in front of me. The run covered only nine yards to the goal line, but as I crossed into the end zone I could not have been more excited if it had been ninety-nine.

Each year brought more involvement and achievements in athletics. Football was my greatest passion but I entered the basketball court, baseball diamond, and track field with equal vigor. My grades steadily improved until at graduation I had a B average. School was not my only center of happiness, for my father had bought a cottage at Baldwin Lake in Michigan. We spent the summers there, fishing, swimming, boating, working, enjoying life each day. I developed a number of close buddies during those five years at Riley. It was hard to believe that our days together as the "Mighty Mite" gang were soon to end. Yet, the ending of one era meant the beginning of another.

There were opportunities for me to attend several different colleges on partial scholarships. But the day I set foot on the campus at Kalamazoo College, I knew where I was going. Nestled into the side of a hill, the wooded quadrangle was rimmed by buildings that contained the classrooms and living quarters of some six hundred students. In spite of the fact that most of my high school friends remained in South Bend to work, or went off to other colleges, I looked forward to the next four years with much eagerness.

College was all I expected it to be—and then some. I had some difficulty with grades the first semester and suffered a separated shoulder as the result of an early football practice. But I quickly adjusted to life away from home. New friends such as roommate "Zeke" Neeser, Ray Glasser, Sam Grow, Roger Gill, "Humph" Hinz, and others, began to fill the void left by former buddies. The athletic arena continued to be the center of attraction, though I enjoyed dating girls and attending various social functions.

My sophomore and junior years at "K" College were dominated by accomplishments in sports and occasional success in campus politics. Coach "Dob" Grow was a deciding influence as I began to develop goals for the future. There still was no place for God in my life, but I had decided to make teaching and coaching my life's work. For the first time I sensed a purpose to what life was about and where I was heading.

Zeke and I had been elected president and vice-president, respectively, of the senior class and I was dating one of the prettiest girls on campus. It was all adding up to a great final year. Having been elected Most Valuable Player in football in my junior year, I awaited the fulfillment offered by the concluding year of my collegiate career. Little did I know that these hopes and dreams would go unfulfilled and my life would take a radical change in course.

POLIO TO THE PRESENT

The reality of what polio had done did not sink in until I had been transferred to Children's Hospital near the University of Notre Dame. As one whose life had revelled in athletics, I found complete paralysis extremely hard to accept. Added to my depressed state of mind was the fact that I had made no provisions to deal with such a crisis. The days and weeks that followed the initial attack seemed empty and endless. I all but gave up on life's having any future.

In January of 1953 I was transferred to Bronson Hospital in Kalamazoo, Michigan, because of its physical therapy program, and it made me nearer to my college friends. It was there that I met the very special young lady who would later become my wife. Theresa Drenth (hereafter known as Tres) and I had no awareness of what the future held, especially on the first day she walked into my room as a special-duty nurse.

The year-and-a-half I spent at Bronson Hospital was a period of mental, emotional, and spiritual change. Perhaps most significant was the spiritual struggle and eventual beginning of my Christian pilgrimage. Tres and others had an influence in bringing me to the point of reevaluating some basic beliefs. I began to come to terms with God. When Christ finally was allowed to become my Lord and Savior, it seemed that my life had made an about-face from my days in high school as an aspiring young athlete.

The therapy I received gave me as much preparation for life ahead as was possible. I was able to use a portable chest respirator which allowed me more freedom of activity than did the confining embrace of the iron lung. I learned to type about thirty-three words a minute on an electric typewriter, tapping the keys with a stick held in my mouth. The total of one year and eleven months between the day I entered Memorial Hospital and the day I left Bronson in a wheelchair, represented both the destruction and rebuilding of my life.

On July 28, 1954, I returned to South Bend and a new start. Tres and I were married in a lovely chapel in South Bend the following October. We knew the future would have disappointments and unique problems, but we also had found a faith in God that encouraged us on to this new life. We lived with my father and cousin for a time, but by January 1956 we were able to have our own home. On October 26, 1957, our daughter Lori was born to complete our family as it now exists.

Many changes have taken place in the daily routine of our lives in sixteen years of marriage. Church involvement and our sense of responsibility in serving Jesus Christ dominate our time and interests. But no small amount of energy has been invested in the home-operated business. It all began with selling magazine subscriptions by telephone. Soon we added greeting cards. Business has increased to the point where, during the fall selling season, we work up to twelve hours a day. Tres handles the telephone, delivers cards, and maintains a somewhat normal household, while I work at the typewriter. Lori, now thirteen, is a vital part of our team effort to accomplish a day's work.

To say this is the sum total of my life to date would be misleading. I have merely given you a bird's-eye view of my life, from past to present. Hopefully you have caught a glimpse of that life like it was. The chapters that follow tell some experiences I've had and philosophies which have developed as the result of my particular circumstance in life. *I'll Walk Tomorrow!* is an earnest effort to relate Jesus Christ as he is to me today!

Chapter 2

Programming Attitudes

How would you answer the question, What must I know to live and die happily? It is a question each person must answer either directly or indirectly, but be assured, there is no avoiding it. Our reply will be influenced by our general outlook on life, and its resulting attitudes.

Several months ago I had the opportunity to speak at a church in Indianapolis. Following the service an elderly man I judged to be in his eighties came up to me. His twinkling eyes and warm smile evidenced the depth and joy of his Christian life. His only comment was, "When we are back home with God, we'll sit down and have a good talk." With a knowing wink, he stuck two dollars in my pocket, turned to two children nearby and filled their hands with pieces of candy. Then he cautiously walked away. Though this encounter was brief, there was no mistaking the view of life he had. His very attitude gave witness to the satisfaction and meaning Jesus Christ had brought into his long life.

TRUE ADVICE?

In contrast to this is an experience Tres and I had with a certain doctor during the early years of our marriage. We sought his advice concerning our home-operated magazine subscription business and general need of income. We were faced with the awareness that financial aid from the National Polio Foundation would soon end, leaving our income far below what was needed. The doctor's suggestion was for my wife to put me in a state hospital (where care would be free), have Tres go to work and live in an apartment. The attitude-revealing comment he concluded with was, "Besides, no two people can be together so much and get along!" It was little surprise to us when we learned that this same doctor was divorced several years later! It would appear that his outlook on marriage produced an attitude that assured the destruction of that relationship.

These two illustrations represent attitudes and a particular view of life. We each have our own vantage point. We see the various aspects of life through our own eyes, influenced by background, environment, and circumstances in which we find ourselves.

Children often are quick to see things as they are. Their attitudes usually are revealed by verbal reaction.

Tres and I visited a pastor and his family in Ohio one particular weekend. When we arrived, Tres proceeded to unload my wheelchair from the rear car seat.

It requires several minutes to unfold the chair, put the detachable pieces in place, and position the sponge pad upon which I sit.

When all was ready, Tres lifted me from the car into the chair. During this time the pastor's five-year-old daughter observed every movement, closely watching each piece of equipment. Not until I had been taken into the house and my portable respirator hooked up did she speak her first words: "Wow! Where did you get that buggy?" My physical condition did not impress her, but in her eyes I had the ultimate in buggies.

A friend of mine who had polio a year before me, had a different kind of reaction. Bill Smoker, also a quadriplegic like me, tells of an experience he had with a young boy. Bill had been pushed to the vestibule following a church service. He was there only a few minutes when he noticed this young boy charging toward him. Without a word the boy doubled his fist, swung, and hit Bill squarely in the chest. He then quickly turned and ran, half crying, half angry.

Bill never did get an explanation of this reaction, but, apparently, the child saw Bill's physical condition as something bad or distasteful. His particular view of Bill's handicap produced a negative reaction.

DIFFERENT PERSPECTIVE

The Apostle Paul came to terms with some views he had when Jesus appeared to him on the road to Damascus. His previous perspective of life produced an attitude that caused Paul to be one of the leading persecutors of Christ's followers. This encounter with Jesus Christ changed Paul's outlook. He saw things differently. The new attitudes were the result of this new view. It was sometime later that Paul made this profound challenge: "Let this mind be in you, which was also in Christ Jesus" (Phil. 2:5). It is here that I have found the answer to the question I first proposed in this chapter. Let me explain more fully by sharing one of the most difficult periods in my life, one that led to a great discovery.

It all began that day in August 1952 when the doctor told me I had polio. It did not scare me, since I had always been healthy and was in good condition for football practice—to begin a week later. My senior year at Kalamazoo College held a great deal of promise. Not only did I expect to excel in sports, but I was anticipating a full social life, and would assume responsibilities of several offices to which I had been elected. Life looked great and I could not believe at that instant anything serious would come from polio.

Two days later I awoke to the rhythmic, mechanical sound of an iron lung. It surrounded my body like a cylindrical cocoon. There I was, dependent upon a metal machine for breath itself, and completely paralyzed from my neck down. My conscious mind would not allow for such reality. I kept thinking, *Not me!*

This couldn't be happening to me! I even remember telling Dob Grow, my football coach, who spent many long hours with me that first week, "I'll be ready to play by the first game!" And I really thought so.

Days began to stretch into weeks and the full realization of what polio had done to me sank in. Suddenly it was obvious that my much-anticipated final year in college was no longer possible. I would not again enjoy the exhilarating thrill of hearing the fans scream as I broke through the line of scrimmage into the open. No longer valid were my dreams of teaching and coaching, of marrying and having a home and family. My outlook on life changed from promise and optimism to discouragement and meaninglessness. My view of life became no larger than the ten-by-twelve-inch mirror hung above my face on the lung.

With the world I had so independently created now destroyed, my perspective of life as a whole produced an attitude of bitterness and resentment. I tried hard to conceal my innermost feelings, but there were times when it was evident to members of my immediate family. It was not uncommon for me to cry from self-pity or to say unkind things to those closest to me. In my mind I lashed out at God though I had not allowed him to be part of my life before. There seemed to be no hope, no escape, and life seemed hardly worth living. My attitudes were being programmed by how I viewed my circumstances.

It was not until after I had been transferred to Bronson Hospital in Kalamazoo, Michigan, that a change began to take place. An intense physical therapy program began to produce results. Being weaned from the iron lung to the portable chest respirator literally brought me a different view. Instead of lying on my back twenty-four hours a day I now could sit up in a chair.

Learning to type on an electric typewriter using a stick placed in my mouth gave me a sense of accomplishment. Each achievement provided a ray of hope. Yet, there was still the feeling of meaninglessness. I knew my life was still completely dependent upon others. Questions like, what can I accomplish? how will I live? will I ever marry? and many more crowded my mind. Life still was without purpose.

During this same period at Bronson Hospital another kind of therapy was going on. Different persons were talking to me about God. Rev. Larry Reynolds, pastor of a south side church in South Bend, drove many 150-mile trips to visit me. Bill and Eddye Lisenko often shared what Christ had done in their lives. Don and June Rice made periodic visits, always having a softly-spoken prayer with me before leaving. Slowly but surely God was beginning to deal with me through these who were faithfully witnessing.

It was also at this time that a nurse by the name of Theresa Drenth came into my life. From the very first meeting, we sensed a special fascination for each other. It was not until almost a year later that the fascination began to develop into a serious relationship. I knew Tres was a Christian. As she and I began to fall in love, the subject of God became more and more a part of our conversations. When the topic of marriage came up, Tres made a statement that caused me to seriously consider my own stance. She said, "I'll give up anything for you except my faith in God."

SEARCH FOR MEANING

I had been searching for meaning in life. Reasoning had failed. Logic only served to confuse the situation. Each direction I turned seemed to lead off into hopelessness—with one exception. It finally occured to me that I really had never given God a chance.

One evening while watching TV alone in my hospital room, I suddenly felt the urge to pray. I had the TV turned off to prevent any distractions. In those moments that followed God seemed real to me for the first time. I knew this was the answer I had been looking for. The searching was over. With no great fanfare and in the quietness of that moment, I asked Jesus Christ to come into my life.

It was as Paul stated in 2 Corinthians 5:17, "Therefore, if any one is in Christ, he is a new creation; the old has passed away, behold, the new has come." This happened to me. My view of life changed almost immediately. Life seemed to matter after all, for I realized God cared. I now had new hope! There was a reason to live!

With each passing year as the "mind of Christ" becomes more a part of me, life is seen as a thrill and adventure with purpose. Attitudes are a direct reflection of my surrender to God's view of myself and my surroundings. Bitterness and resentment are no longer part of my outlook.

A computer's responses are the result of the program it has been fed. Human responses to life's experiences are the result of what is allowed to impress our minds. As Jesus influences our way of thinking, we will increasingly respond as he would. Our attitudes are being programmed constantly as we select and determine those values each feels are important.

To live and die happily a person first must establish a relationship with God. This is available to all, no matter who we are or in what circumstance we find ourselves. This relationship is realized through Jesus Christ.

Chapter *3*

Born Free

If someone had asked me prior to the time I had polio, "What is the worst thing that could possibly happen to you?" my most likely reply would have been, "To be completely paralyzed!"

That response is not difficult to understand when you realize my heart and mind were centered on sports. My physical well-being was important at that particular time in my life. Goals such as making first-string on the football or basketball team, being able to perform better than the next guy to keep my position were given priority in all things.

Paralysis, to me then, represented a stigma on life, a confinement and restriction, a lack of freedom. It implied dependence and that was low on my list of "life's desires." My physical abilities and accomplishments bought freedom and independence. I did not want anything to happen to that!

The last several years there has been much talk about "doing your own thing" or more recently just "do it." There seems to be a constant struggle for people to feel free, to do as they please, to avoid restrictions society places upon them. The search is on to find ways and means to such freedoms. Some today apparently believe the answer is in drugs. Others turn to sex, defiance of authority, alcohol, materialism. Yet, this is really nothing new. It has been a desire of each generation throughout the ages. Each of us has this inner desire to feel free and independent.

LIFE REALLY BEGINS

As I approach the age when some say life begins: forty, it occurs to me that half of my life has been lived under normal, healthy, physical conditions while the other half has been lived in a wheelchair, paralyzed, dependent on others for breath and food. Strange as it may seem to many, it has been only since I had polio and accepted Jesus Christ as Lord and Savior that I have felt genuine freedom, truly released from inner conflicts that influence attitudes and actions. John records Jesus as saying in chapter 8, verse 36, "So if the Son makes you free, you will be free indeed." This has been my experience.

One of my acquaintances in recent years has been "Cal," a handicapped young man with a crippled right arm and deformed hand. Upon meeting Cal you would first be impressed by the broad smile and sparkling shiny eyes against his black face. Your next response would be to shake hands as he pushes his right hand toward you. Chances are you would not be shocked or uneasy for his friendly manner and lack of self-consciousness put you immediately at ease.

Cal, through practice and hard work, has acquired the skillful use of his right arm to supplement his good left arm. But more than that, he has been set free from his handicap by his attitude and acceptance of the misfortune. The outwardly happy expression of his personality reflects his inner satisfaction.

In no small way most of us strive to find freedom from whatever restricts or confines us. Some find marriage to be a monumental restriction when it actually is an opportunity to be free to express and experience love in all its depth. Others find their occupations confining when these tasks should mean freedom to create and contribute to the world around them. Attitudes toward others because of race or religion or unusual circumstances can be as confining as a jail cell. To be released from prejudice of any kind will free our minds which in turn will allow us to be the kind of person God has in mind.

Tres and I have many opportunities to meet people as we travel on occasional speaking dates. In many instances we all-too-well recognize the well-intentioned expression of sympathy or the familiar sad smile when persons see me sitting in a wheelchair. Often in contrast are the children we meet. They always delight me.

On one particular occasion I had just been lifted up a flight of stairs by three husky men into the foyer of a church. A bright-faced girl of about seven came rushing toward me, wide-eyed, laid her hands on my arm, and said, "What happened to you?" Not waiting for a reply, she began to investigate the marvelous gadgets on the wheelchair. With a brief touch here, a glance there, she noticed how the leg rests adjust, the arms detach, and the chair can be collapsed. As her mother led her away I heard her ask, "Mom, can I get one of those?"

The difference in response is that some see the negative side of the circumstances: the fact that I cannot walk, cannot shake hands, cannot breathe without mechanical help. Children often see only the uniqueness, the advantages. This has illustrated to me the fact that how we see ourselves directly affects our freedom to become the persons we really can be.

During high school and college days, I thought I was on my way to becoming my own man. I figured I had control of life and was directing my own destiny. God was not needed. I could captain my own ship. I saw my life as the center of activities, with the rest of the world revolving around it. In short, I was my own captive limited by self and selfish desires. Life was neither deeper nor broader than the values I established for myself. When polio destroyed those values I found myself hopelessly void of meaning.

A BETTER WAY

Jesus, I discovered several years later, already had suggested a better way for life to operate at peak efficiency. When we attempt to run things our way exclusively, when we try to save our lives, we end up losing them. When we yield control to Christ, then we have life in all its freedom and fullness. Then, and only then, can we begin to shed the shackles of self and the servants of self: greed, pride, prejudice, envy, jealousy, fear. As Jesus Christ becomes a reality, as the Holy Spirit begins to share our life, then we can be set free to become, to do, and to be the man, woman, young person we desire.

Booker T. Washington experienced just such freedom, as indicated by his statement, "I will not permit any man to narrow and degrade my soul by making me hate him." No man can truly achieve this kind of freedom without having Jesus set him free. God had established within Booker Washington a much higher standard that allowed him the freedom to act toward another out of brotherly love.

There is no situation or circumstance in life from which we cannot be set free. Our actions often may be restricted, our bodies may be confined at times, our jobs and personal involvements may hold us within boundaries. But we can have the freedom to experience life in its entirety and to its fullest meaning. Life holds much more value to me now than ever before because

Jesus Christ has established its worth. I am free from my physical handicap because God sees it as a positive factor: something that has added to my life. No longer can I say, "Being paralyzed is the worst thing that could happen to me!" I was born free when I met Christ!

This freedom is available to everyone, no matter who you are, where you are, or in what circumstance you find yourself.

Chapter *4*

Dialogue with the World

My first opportunity to witness for Jesus Christ was a flop! It happened a week after I had made the decision to accept Christ into my life. A college buddy had come to visit me one evening in the hospital. We were talking about trivialities when he suddenly said, "What do you think about God?" My immediate reaction was shock, for we had never discussed such matters before. It even sounded a little strange to hear the word *god* used in a way other than an expression of ill feelings. Many of my friends up to then would not have been caught dead talking kindly about God.

By the time I regained my composure, I heard myself saying, "Oh, I think there probably is a God, but that's all I know about it."

His response was, "Yeh, it's sort of so-so with me, too." We then quickly dropped the subject and went on to more important topics, such as, who would win the World Series.

Later that evening when I was alone again, I felt sick at heart. Like I had betrayed a good friend. It was somewhat puzzling at the time to understand why I had such feelings. I had not been educated to the idea yet that Christians are also witnesses. But it was apparent that an opportunity had been available for me to share my newfound faith in Jesus Christ.

HELP FOR WITNESSING

Failure to witness on this first occasion, however, has been a help to me in several ways ever since. It was like being thrown from a horse for the first time. You pick yourself up, dust off your trousers, and prepare with apprehension to climb back into the saddle. Once you have regained control, assurance and confidence quickly assert themselves. God used my failure to help establish even more firmly that spark of faith I had confessed a short week before. In that moment of guilt I recognized the reality of God. I knew Jesus had become part of me.

To witness means to tell forth. More specifically it is to share truths from the depths of our life experiences and convictions. Some may think the only effective way this can be done is by the spoken or printed word. But someone has said, "What you are speaks so loudly that I can't hear what you say." The point is, we witness in every way there is communication. It is obvious that when our *actions* prove to be sincere and honest, it will go a long way to support that what we *say* is true.

Several years ago, a family from Puerto Rico moved into a house across the street from our family. Because they spoke Spanish and little else, they often had a difficult time trying to communicate. Lori decided one day to try to talk with the six-year-old boy. It was hopeless in spite of their attempt to make signs with their hands. A few days later Lori found stored in the closet two books which she thought might solve the communication barrier. The books contained pictures with appropriate Spanish words and matching words in English. From that day on it did not take the children long to communicate ideas to each other.

This achievement in communication was the result of not just saying the words but seeing their meanings. Dialogue often breaks down when we fail to convey meanings. To witness is to use more than words, it is communicating living pictures and images. Our actions and attitudes present a picture of truth that gives credence to our words.

Certainly there are many ways to witness. There are those who obtain results using the hard-sell or bold approach. There is a time to knock on doors, to hand out tracts, and to tell every saleslady or businessman that Jesus died for them. On the other hand, others find more success through serving. Visiting shut-ins, praying with the sick, providing food and clothes for the needy, are ways of saying, "God loves you!" Jesus himself said, "But if any one has the world's goods and sees his brother in need, yet closes his heart against him, how does God's love abide in him? Little children, let us not love in word or speech but in deed and in truth" (1 John 3:17-18).

NO SINGLE METHOD

I am convinced that no one method is the only way to witness. All have merit. But over the long haul I have found the most effective witness comes as we encounter experiences daily. It is a matter of being opportunists in the best sense of the word. The Apostle Paul's philosophy was, "I have become all things to all men, that I might by all means save some" (1 Corinthians 9:22). Each situation we encounter presents an opportunity to not just tell others what God can do, but literally to show them. Educators know that the best teaching method is to show and tell.

Tres and I became friends of Clyde and Mary Haney while they were living in South Bend. Some fifteen years ago Clyde was hospitalized because of a severe problem with alcohol. Near the end of the almost two years he spent in the hospital, Clyde was led into a tremendous conversion experience. He recognized Jesus Christ as the answer to his problem. A short time later he was released to return home to Mary and their three children.

One of the interesting aspects of Clyde's conversion has to do with those who were able to witness to him. Some persons from Alcoholics Anonymous, who had gone through a similar experience and understood his problem, most effectively reached Clyde. He was able to see with his own eyes that Jesus really would make the difference because of what he had done in the lives of those who were sharing the Good News. They were *showing* Clyde what God can do, not just *telling* him!

TANGIBLE INTANGIBLE

It was much the same in my case. I was not influenced so much by those who visited me once and said things like, "Jesus died for you," or, "God loves the sinner." Those who took the time to visit and share from their life experiences had the greatest effect on my ultimate decision to accept Christ as Savior. For in those who made that effort, I recognized a genuine concern for me as a person. It was not a duty or chore but, obviously, an act of love and deep interest. I felt that they would not take the time to drive hundreds of miles, in some instances, to tell what God had done in their lives if it were not a reality.

In contrast to those who took the time to share from their experiences was a zealous young man we had occasion to encounter. Tres and I attended services during a two-week tent revival meeting. Because of my wheelchair, it was necessary for me to sit in the aisle. One of the ushers was a young man who seemed to take more interest in us than he did in others who attended each evening. He always found a place near the front for us to sit. Following the message one particular night, this young man apparently was overcome by the desire to see me accept Christ.

We were sitting with heads bowed when suddenly I felt someone grab the back of my wheelchair and shove me toward the altar. The locked wheels hindered him not. Sawdust flew as the wheels dug into the ground. When we skidded to a stop at the altar rail, I glanced over my shoulder and saw the usher's gleaming face, a smile spread from ear to ear. His quick explanation was, "You need Jesus Christ in your life." When I informed him that Jesus was already a reality to me, his face turned to an expression of bewilderment if not a tinge of disappointment.

Most of us can appreciate the enthusiasm of such a witness, but there was no way to force me into such a decision. Christ never forced himself upon others. He simply conveyed his message through words and deeds. There is no trick or sham to the fact that God loves us —it is an experience of reality. This message and experience of reality can best be shared through the whole of life, not just in part. Most people we meet are not interested merely in what we say about our religion. They also want to see what we are doing with it!

The four Gospels reveal Jesus as One who ministered as opportunities and occasions presented themselves. From the woman at the well to Lazarus, from the woman accused of adultery to the healing of the ten lepers, Christ used each encounter to tell who he was and why he had come. If there is a valid method or pattern to follow, it is to be found here.

WITNESS IN LIFE

The greatest opportunities we Christians have are in the midst of life's involvements. Our witness is as unique as our set of friends, acquaintances, relatives, neighbors, and community. It is as relevant as each encounter. It is as meaningful as we recognize the needs of those with whom we are involved. Each man, woman, young person, or child who has accepted Jesus has a ministry. A ministry only each individual can perform, because he is who he is! In the Sermon on the Mount, Jesus makes two profound statements: "You are the salt of the earth" and "You are the light of the world" (Matthew 5:13-14). Recognizing this responsibility, we can begin dialogue with the world.

God has allowed me a unique tool with which to witness. My paralysis, the wheelchair, and respirator all provide me with opportunities to reveal the love of God. When others see the difference Jesus Christ has made in my life in spite of these handicaps, hopefully they not only hear what I am saying but see it as well.

Dr. Ewald Wolfram once told me, "Witnessing is like a water faucet. Unless you turn it on you won't get the water!" Our lives are much like that faucet. The Lord supplies the "rivers of living water" but it is our responsibility to allow the flow of his love to be expressed through us. Jesus Christ is counting on you and me!

Chapter **5**

Follow the Yellow Brick Road

In the story "The Wizard of Oz," Dorothy and her companions: the Scarecrow, Tin-Man, and Lion, were given the advice to "Follow the yellow brick road" if they wanted to reach their destination. Obviously the path we determine to follow throughout life is not so clearly marked. In fact, there seem to be many paths to follow in every experience we encounter, each saying, "Go this way." The decisions we make will to a great degree depend upon the principles and standards we allow to guide our life.

CHRISTIAN GUIDANCE

We who have accepted Jesus Christ into our life have a particular advantage. God already has established guidelines for us to follow. The problem is that we often do not bother to read the road signs. It is difficult at times to know upon what to base our determinations. Yet, if there is a key to the Christian life, it is in being able to determine God's way. If each

Christian is to live his life to the fullest extent and with the greatest meaning, he must arrive at a method to satisfy his own mind about what God desires.

SEARCH FOR GOD'S WILL

Tres and I went through a critical period of trying to determine God's will prior to our marriage. There were many decisions to make even before we got to the one big decision. In every case the answers were not easy. Tres had to determine whether or not she wanted to give her life to someone she would have to help daily in every way. It would be a matter of feeding, dressing, and providing companionship beyond what is normally expected of a wife. I had to decide how I could provide for a wife and be a contributor to a normal family-life situation.

Together we had to be sure our love was strong enough to weather not only the normal adjustments of marriage but the problems we would face because of my physical handicap. Attempting to discover God's will became our primary goal. Yet, this was not clearly spelled out at first.

We began by praying that God would reveal his will to us. Tres had known the Lord longer and better, so I relied heavily upon her insights. I had made my decision for Christ only a short time before and I was a little unsure of my prayers. But in faith I sought God's leading.

We also began to discuss as many aspects of our future together as we could foresee. It was a matter of trying to understand that our marriage would be different in some respects. It was important that we know the prospects of successfully operating a business in a home under such circumstances. We had to investigate ways and means of travel. From the sources available to us advice was sought on the unanswered questions in our minds. In short, we attempted to answer and solve beforehand as many problems as we could.

I was a nervous young man the night I finally popped the question to Tres. There still were some unanswered questions and we had encountered some discouraging advice from a few friends and doctors. But I felt right in asking her to marry me. The affirmative response she gave only served to confirm my conviction. She also had reached the conclusion that this was what God desired, for she had been seeking to know his mind above all else. Together we had been able to discern God's will through the confidence and assurance we felt in entering into this lifelong relationship.

FAITH AND LOGIC

When making such a determination as God's will, I find it necessary to put all related ingredients together. The Holy Spirit living in our life provides the source of impressions and desires in line with the

Lord's wishes. Logic and understanding also add greatly to the overall considerations in making such decisions. I do not believe we can divorce completely from seeking God's will what our better judgment tells us. We were created with both a mind and the power of reasoning. Each must be used.

In contrast to the more difficult decision of marriage, Tres and I had another experience a few years later. When I was released from Bronson Hospital in Kalamazoo, we had returned to South Bend to live in a rented house with my father. It was not long after that when we began to entertain thoughts of having our own home. At first it seemed almost impossible to us. Our magazine subscription business was only a year old and not yet very productive. The only other source of income was what the Polio Foundation was paying Tres to care for me. Neither source was guaranteed or adequate and we had no other assets except a six-year-old Ford.

We began at the point experience had already taught us: we prayed to know God's mind about such an undertaking. We were confident the way would open to solve the problems if we were to have our own home.

Things started to happen almost at once. Mr. Vernon Hazzard, Director of the local Goodwill Industries, gave me a part-time job working with the Women's Auxiliary. During the fall of 1955 our magazine business doubled and we had added Christmas greeting cards to our sales line. These at least were signs to us of a financial go-ahead.

The next revelation came as we were searching the "House for Sale" ads in the newspaper. I noticed a salesman's name that had a familiar look to it. Upon inquiring, I learned the salesman was the former Director of Admissions at Kalamazoo College, Bob Braithwaite. In a conversation with Bob later that week, after we had discussed old times, I told him of our interest in finding a home. The following week Bob called back to say he had found just the house for us, on East Chippewa Avenue. When Tres and I drove over to see it I think we both began to sense God's influence in the whole affair. There was no "yellow brick road" to follow but the path seemed clearly marked.

BRIDGES TO CROSS

Though it all seemed so logical at this point, there still were some bridges to cross. Because of my physical handicap and the fact that we were newly self-employed, we were unable to obtain an FHA loan to buy the house. This was solved when the owners of the house suggested that we assume their mortgage; that is, pay them the money they had invested to date and take over their loan. We did have to borrow additional money for the down payment but this was made available through my mother and stepfather. Once the house was bought we still needed furniture and appliances, both of which we had none. Somehow even this had a solution as the result of the increased profits from our business and careful budgeting. When we moved into our own home in January of 1956, we knew with certainty that this, too, was God's choice.

EXPERIENCE GIVES INSIGHT

These two early experiences in our married life have provided us with a source of insight into seeking God's will throughout each new experience. Though the circumstances and decisions to be made are different, still there is the familiar pattern of praying, seeking, reasoning, and determining. Some decisions are difficult, while others are relatively easy. Included in our sixteen years of marriage are periods of indecision and wrong decisions.

But we have sought God's way in such matters as friendships, church involvement, witnessing, income opportunities, giving advice on marriage problems, raising a daughter, and on the list goes. To be sure, I have not found a foolproof way to determine God's will. I am convinced, however, that he uses many ways to communicate his desires to us. The effectiveness each of us has is the result of our ability to listen to him and apply reasoning to the facts at hand.

It also has been my experience that God at times provides a multiple choice. There have been occasions when I was firmly convinced that a decision I made was absolutely correct. In retrospect, however, it was easy to see that any one of several choices would have been right in God's sight. This has assured me that the Lord's will is not always a narrow channel of decisions but rather a wide experience of learning to live life abundantly, in completeness and fullness. I believe his will leads us in paths that are meaningful and have everlasting influence on our lives to better equip us day by day.

There are three bases upon which to build our communication with God if we truly wish to do his will. They are to (1) have an understanding of what God requires of us, (2) know that God has our best interest at heart, (3) know that he will supply our needs in order to fulfill his will.

KNOWING WHAT GOD REQUIRES

Generally speaking, we can come to an understanding of what God requires of us by praying, studying the Bible and other inspirational sources, being aware of and becoming involved in the needs of people around us, and remaining viable to the instruction and advice of others. In the book of Micah, there is a passage that has meant much to me in this area: "He hath showed thee, O man, what is good; and what doth the Lord require of thee, but to do justly, and to love mercy, and to walk humbly with thy God" (6:8).

In these three statements Micah covers the essential areas of all of life's experiences and encounters. Unless we are willing to attempt to assimilate these attitudes and actions into our life, it will be most difficult to determine God's will. Surely it is obvious that this *is* the Lord's will. Then can we do less than make these our primary aims? It encompasses our relationship with neighbors, friends, relatives, the poor, the rich, people of other races, even wives or husbands. It involves our attitudes toward and actual involvement with needs as we encounter them. And, finally, it requires an active relationship with God: we should *walk* with God, not *stand*.

GOD HAS OUR INTEREST AT HEART

Greg Parker was one of my coaches when I attended Riley High School. Greg coached the football and basketball B teams which included boys in the tenth and eleventh grades. Those of you who are or at one time were athletic have had the unique experience of performing practice drills hour after hour. Greg was an expert in this category and I must admit there were days when I thought it was a waste of time. We would rather have played a game, shot baskets, or caught passes. But as I went on to varsity and college sports, I began to realize just how important those years of basic drills were. It also made me recognize that Greg Parker had our best interest at heart. He wanted each of us to become as fine an athlete as ability and effort would allow. My achievements in sports certainly would not have been the same without those years under Greg.

In a very similar way I feel God has our interest at heart. We each have periods when we wonder *Why did God allow this?* or *Why did things turn out this way?* There were times when I asked these questions because of my physical handicap. Nevertheless, I now am confident God wants each experience—good or bad—to add to the stature of our lives.

Jesus Christ had a similar question in mind when he prayed in the Garden while his disciples waited. Jesus had asked that the cup of suffering and death might pass from him, but God had other plans. It was then that Christ followed with the all-important "nevertheless, not my will but thine be done." There is no need here of a dissertation on the implications of this molding together of two wills into one.

GOD WILL SUPPLY OUR NEEDS

A missionary once told me, "If God gives you a task, he will supply the means to accomplish it." I would amplify that by saying that God will supply the resources in each life to accomplish his will. The only difficulty is that we sometimes fail to recognize or use his resources.

As a young mischievous boy of ten, I once pinned a neighbor's car horn. This was one of the more daring pranks boys pulled at Halloween time. I vividly remember how I placed a stick into the steering wheel, letting it press against the horn. Before I had a chance to turn and run, the porch light blazed on and out the door rushed the car's owner. I quickly ran between two dark houses and across the backyard, but I knew a four-foot fence stood in my path of escape. I had never been able to jump that fence before, but that night I bounded over it with inches to spare. I had found a source of strength out of fright.

Deuteronomy 31:8 records Moses telling Joshua in front of all Israel: "It is the Lord who goes before you; he will be with you, he will not fail you or forsake you; do not fear or be dismayed." This applies to you and me as well. When we find ourselves in a difficult position or attempting to make an important decision, we can consciously realize that God is there, too. When we do we will find a reservoir of strength and insight untapped by any other frame of mind. Even as I discovered new strength from being afraid I would be caught, so the awareness of God's presence provides a faith and confidence otherwise unknown.

Once you have made these three convictions your own, God's will then becomes not so much a "going from one experience or decision to another" but an instinctive subconscious desire to make your will his will. At this point we can begin to live our lives as Christ lived his. The decisions that continually confront us become less difficult to make as we learn of and yield to God's presence in our lives.

DIFFICULT DECISIONS

Two close friends of ours at one stage in their lives faced a most difficult decision. Don and June Rice were married while attending Anderson College. Upon graduating they moved to South Bend where Don acquired a good job with the Studebaker Corporation. Within a short time they were able to buy their own home and were well on the way to financial independence and security. It was not long, however, until Don began to have thoughts about a different occupation. Because of his college preparation in the area of Christian education, he began to consider entering the teaching profession.

To accomplish this meant some sacrifices. It would require Don's returning to college for graduate work to obtain a teaching certificate. It also meant both Don and June would have to give up their jobs and sell their home. They began to pray as well as evaluate the implications of making such a decision. As Don recounted the experience to me recently, he told how he became convinced that Christians were needed in the field of education. He said that after months of considering such a step, it finally boiled down to his question, "Is teaching really what I want to do with my life?" The forthcoming answer was yes and the decision was made.

God's will had been sought and followed, not be-cause of a crash prayer program or because it was written in the clouds. The decision was the fruition of two lives given to Jesus Christ many years earlier. It was the end result of allowing God to be permanently resident in their lives. Because their communication with God was a continuing, active process, Don and June were able to reach a decision in line with his. Upon their return to South Bend after graduate work, Don not only entered the teaching profession but has since become principal of one of the larger junior high schools in the area.

For me, seeking God's will is not so much a matter of looking for unusual signs, but is a conscious awareness of God at work in my life. There are no magic formulas or roads painted yellow. His will is made known in proportion to my efforts to listen. My ability to really hear is the result of consistent prayer life, earnest seeking, and the power to reason. To discover and walk in God's will, then, is the key to satisfying, meaningful Christian life!

Chapter **6**

God Answers

I have asked God to heal me. Though I am still paralyzed, he has indeed answered my prayer. You may consider my remarks a form of double-talk or, at best, you would like an explanation of why I am so convinced.

To be sure, we are accustomed to considering the complete restoration of the body as healing. I have been told many times by Christians that God wants to heal me. There seems to be little doubt in their minds that if your heart is right and you have sufficient faith, God will restore the body.

I SOUGHT FOR HEALING

During the early part of my Christian life, about seventeen years ago, I felt somewhat the same. On one occasion Tres and I attended faith-healing services every night for two weeks. I was prayed for, along with others, each evening. It was at this time that I had also written to Oral Roberts asking him to pray for my healing as well. I was convinced that God should and would restore my body to its normal state of health. My daily Bible reading was centered on scriptures that had to do with Jesus healing those who were sick or paralyzed. All outward evidence seemed to support my idea. Besides, I wanted to be healed in body in the worst way. I had thoughts of again turning my efforts to athletics.

The fact that I was not healed the way I desired, frustrated me. It did not seem fair since I was trying so hard to achieve the proper frame of mind and spirit. I was praying, searching the scriptures, and other persons were equally concerned on my behalf. The question in my mind was, *Why is God not answering my prayers?*

GLIMMER OF LIGHT

The first glimmer of light came when I ran across a passage of Scripture in 2 Corinthians. Apparently the Apostle Paul had a physical problem. I read in chapter 12, verses 7-11, how earnestly Paul sought healing for his affliction: "And to keep me from being too elated by the abundance of revelations, a thorn was given me in the flesh, a messenger of Satan, to harass me, to keep me from being too elated. Three times I besought the Lord about this, that it should leave me; but he said to me, 'My grace is sufficient for you, for my power is made perfect in weakness.' I will all the more gladly boast of my weaknesses, that the power of Christ may rest upon me. For the sake of Christ, then, I am content with weaknesses, insults, hardships, persecutions, and calamities; for when I am weak, then I am strong."

Paul had asked God to heal him. He wanted to be restored, to be free of the physical difficulty. Yet, God did not eliminate the "thorn" from the life of this great man of faith. It then occurred to me that perhaps there is something else, another answer, besides physical healing. I began to see healing from a new perspective. The thought was born, *Is God saying that his grace is sufficient for me, too?*

As I began to lift my eyes above my own circumstances and desires, I realized there were many afflicted persons who had served God but who had not been physically restored. Charles W. Naylor wrote many inspiring gospel songs while confined to bed and in severe pain. Fanny Crosby, though blind from birth, composed more than five thousand hymns during her lifetime, sometimes as many as seven a day. There have been many such as Helen Keller who lived their lives for God while physically handicapped. The scores of Negro Spirituals were born out of the depths of despair and torment. As I saw the love and mercy of God in such living examples, it became clear to me that healing could take place in another way.

NEW REVELATION

This new revelation made me realize that in my case the search for healing was somewhat selfish. I had overlooked the possibility that God could use me more effectively in a wheelchair. My desire was to be restored to a normal life again. I wanted to run, work with my hands, feed myself, take a shower, and even mow the yard. Until then, I had not considered that God may have a better way.

It was in the midst of this transitional period that Bill Lisenko made me face the idea that God has his own timing and way of healing. During those years following my conversion Bill spent many evenings relating one Bible story after another. It was like having a living commentary for a friend. The compassion of Jesus and his many miracles of healing became alive. Bill made me aware of God's love and mercy for each of us as individuals. He also sowed the first seeds in my mind that eventually led to an important discovery. That is, God's healing power extends beyond the physical. This was a vital link in my struggle to understand why I had not been physically healed.

In looking back over the years to my early beginning as a Christian, I can now see with certain clarity that God has healed me. Yes, I am still physically paralyzed from the neck down and I live life on four wheels. But the grace God has healed me with is more than sufficient to make my handicap a real blessing. From this particular vantage point, I would like to share several conclusions uncovered in my searchings.

HEALING MUST BE SOUGHT

First, there is only one prerequisite to healing. It must be sought! Jesus himself said it this way: "Ask, and it will be given you; seek, and you will find; knock, and it will be opened to you. For everyone who asks receives, and he who seeks finds, and to him who knocks it will be opened" (Matthew 7:7-8).

It has become quite evident to me that you cannot *earn* healing, for it is a gift from God. He bestows this gift upon us as he does salvation, but we must seek it. Healing cannot be forced for it comes in God's way and time.

One splendid example of this is illustrated in the book *A Man Called Peter*. Catherine Marshall, widow of the great Scottish preacher, tells of her struggles with tuberculosis. For over two years, during most of which she was confined to bed, Catherine continually asked God to heal her of this disease. At one point, she relates, she attempted to correct all the unkindness and injustice she had caused, thinking that God was holding something against her. After many months of searching and seeking to bring her life up to the proper level, she finally had to give up in despair. In utter defeat she concluded, "Lord, if you want me to remain like this, here I am. I am yours!" It was then that God touched her body and physically restored her.

There is no way to win or merit healing from God. The many incidents of Jesus healing the sick and the crippled in the New Testament reveal that there were those who barely knew who he really was. At best, some had heard he performed miracles, but to claim an abundance of faith or a Godly life would be less than factual. To be certain, Jesus acknowledged the importance of faith. In Matthew 9:22 he says, "Take heart, daughter; your faith has made you well." But even the greatest amount of faith can only carry us to the point of God's touch. It is for him to extend his healing power as it best suits our total life.

We need to ask, but we cannot demand. We should seek, but we cannot earn. To knock is to extend in faith our desire for God's touch upon our life.

GOD DOES HEAL TODAY

Second, God does heal our bodies and minds. To say or even suggest that miracles of physical healing no longer happen today is to miss one of the meaningful relationships between God and man.

I witnessed the healing of two teen-agers deaf from birth. In prayer God was asked to perfect their hearing. In one swift moment they experienced God's healing hand. Their hearing was given them. For the very first time they heard sounds. I have seen others rise from wheelchairs, discard crutches in an instant. One friend told her experience of being healed of a tumor. Another related her healing from tuberculosis. A church member, disabled in an accident, said to us,

"I know God has healed me, but I don't know why!" On and on go the real-life evidences of God at work touching lives and restoring them to normal.

Within the past two years I was unfortunate enough to contract the so-called "Hong Kong" flu virus. From it I developed pneumonia and had to enter the hospital. Xrays verified that my lungs were partially filled with fluid. It is serious enough to have pneumonia under normal conditions but, because I require a respirator to breathe, it was much more dangerous.

Tres and I prayed that the Lord would undertake my healing of this severe cold complication. Others also were praying on my behalf.

I had been admitted to the hospital on a Thursday. On Saturday the doctor ordered more Xrays. The following day I was told that my lungs were clear and normal and I could go home within the next two days. Certainly the new modern medicines helped, but even the doctor was amazed at the speed of my recovery. God did indeed work his miracle of healing.

The reality of the power of God to heal today is no different than in the days when Jesus walked the dusty roads restoring sight to the blind, health to broken and crippled bodies, clarity of mind to the mentally distressed.

GOD'S GRACE IN HEALING

Third, God's grace heals. G. Campbell Morgan refers to grace as God's activity toward us and in us.

One dictionary defines it as unmerited divine assistance given man for his regeneration or sanctification.

Eugenia Price speaks of grace as God's intention toward us carried out completely in Jesus Christ.

In each definition we quickly recognize the idea that grace is God reaching into our lives. When he does, he adds that source of strength that enables us to conquer any difficult circumstance in which we find ourselves. God, involved in our life, overcomes and uses the difficulties which we, by ourselves, cannot defeat.

I have found it so in my life. Though I have not been physically healed, God has allowed me to live a most satisfying, complete life. I have not only found joy and purpose, I have discovered significant usefulness in my circumstances. The opportunities to serve and be productive are limitless. In short, I no longer sense the hopelessness of a paralyzed body, for God has healed me by his grace!

The Amplified New Testament enlarges on this point in 2 Corinthians 12:9a, "But he said to me, My grace —My favor and loving-kindness and mercy—are enough for you, [that is, sufficient against any danger and to enable you to bear the trouble manfully]; for my strength and power are made perfect—fulfilled and completed and show themselves most effective—in [your] weakness."

This healing power of grace is just as much an answer to prayer as is physical restoration. It is God at work within us to effect his will. The Apostle Paul found it true in his own life.

GOD'S GRACE A MYSTERY

Throughout our lives there are many occasions on which we will petition the Lord for healing, for our own needs or in behalf of others. The way God responds is at times difficult to understand, but it is here that we must learn to trust. One couple Tres and I had opportunity to meet told us about just such an experience.

Their five-year-old child became ill. After a number of examinations the doctor finally gave them the sad news. The child had leukemia. The couple's first reaction was shock, then fear and desperation.

What parent cannot understand the feeling of anguish over a child who is ill? But in a circumstance that is all but hopeless, anguish reaches the point of torment. In this instance the parents were Christians, and they instinctively turned to God. They prayed fervently for their child to be healed. Everything they knew to do, they did, but the child grew steadily worse. It became difficult for them to sleep at night or to think about anything but the welfare of their child. They had reached the breaking point. Wrought with fear and in despair they prayed, "Lord, we give our child to you. Not our will but thine be done!"

In answer to this prayer, the couple later stated, came their first sense of God's assurance, and peace of mind. Their anxiety was relieved, simply because they had decided to put their complete trust in God.

Their young child died several weeks later. Though theirs was the normal hurt, and deep loneliness, they experienced the inner strength of God's presence. Their trust in God had turned pending tragedy into a significant spiritual enlightenment. They had no doubt that their child was with God.

When we hear such stories, we normally react with sympathy. Rightly so, for we see life and death through human eyes, limited by finite minds. God's perspective is different. Isaiah 55:8-9 states, "For my thoughts are not your thoughts, neither are your ways my ways, says the Lord. For as the heavens are higher than the earth, so are my ways higher than your ways and my thoughts than your thoughts." How can we help but trust God who works for our best in his thoughts and in his ways!

God will touch our lives. We may not always recognize the touch, for often we fail to trust. But ask of him what you will. Petition the Lord for your needs. Seek his healing. God will answer, in his way and in his time. Of this I am certain for he has answered my life's prayer for healing.

Chapter 7

What Handicap?

What comes to your mind when you hear the word *handicap*? Most likely you think of a physical impairment of one sort or another. A physical problem often is most obvious and usually results in restriction of what is called normal activity. A mental handicap also would fit into this category, but that is about the extent of the generally accepted definition of the word.

WRONG IMPRESSIONS

Before I had polio I was one of those persons who regard handicapped individuals as being less than normal. It even depressed me to be around such persons. When polio entered the picture of my life, I struggled with this preconceived idea while adjusting to my paralysis. Years later I still refused to use the word handicap in connection with my situation. I preferred the word disabled. It did not seem to have the same bad implications in my mind.

I have learned that many persons have similar feelings toward a person physically or mentally handicapped. A sort of uneasy, uncomfortable feeling. Perhaps many of these ideas come from years ago when handicapped people were looked down upon. They were often uneducated because of their inability to attend school or because of the bad effect authorities thought they would have on more normal children. Some families, out of embarrassment or fear of public scorn, attempted to hide relatives who were handicapped. In times past some afflicted persons were even put to death because it was thought that Satan possessed them. Many written accounts tell of how inhumanly the mentally retarded were treated in dungeons and so-called snake-pits. Is it any wonder that there still are misconceptions about the handicapped today, after such a history?

IDEAS ARE CHANGING

From my own point of view, I feel these straw men are rapidly being overcome. Education is available to all in one form or another today and there really is no reason for a person to be without it. Many new aids have been developed in recent years that help even the most severe physical impairment. Transportation no longer is the problem it once was and many new building codes for public buildings make provisions for users of wheelchairs and crutches. Generally speaking, progress has made the mechanical side of living much easier for those with physical limitations. A physically or mentally handicapped person is accepted in society with less reservation today than ever before. Many limitations no longer need to be considered the handicap they once were. In fact, I believe the word *handicap* in reality implies more than we are normally educated to think.

MANY ARE HANDICAPPED

Today, the word handicap is coming into proper perspective. Traditionally it has been connected with a physical or mental disability, but I see it extending into all areas of life. There are those who have personality handicaps. Some find old age—or youth—to be a handicap. Others may be handicapped by fear, or inferiority, or lack of education. A wife or husband can be a handicap to her/his mate. Each time we directly or indirectly teach a child prejudice based on the color of a man's skin or economic status, we are in a very real sense handicapping that child. In other words, I believe a handicap to be anything that limits us from fulfilling what God intended our lives to be!

Moses of the Old Testament certainly was one of the strong leaders of history. God used him to lead the Hebrew people out of the land of Egypt to the Promised Land. But there was a brief struggle at the time God commissioned Moses to undertake the task. Moses apparently felt he could not speak well enough to be such a leader. The record states, "But Moses said to the Lord, 'Oh, my Lord, I am not eloquent, either heretofore or since thou hast spoken to thy servant; but I am slow of speech and of tongue'" (Exodus 4:10). Moses had imposed a handicap upon himself because of a lack of confidence to speak to other people.

With Jeremiah it was his youth. Note his reply to God's call: "Ah, Lord God! Behold, I do not know how to speak, for I am only a youth" (Jer. 1:6). He was about to allow age to handicap his service to God. The Apostle Peter was momentarily handicapped by fear of persecution when he denied Jesus Christ three times in a brief period.

In each of these illustrations we discover by reading the context that their handicaps were overcome as they responded to God. It is that way in each of our lives if we will but recognize it. All too often, however, we fail to look to God in our attempts to overcome handicaps, whatever they are.

Over the years that I have been paralyzed, I have met many with physical impairments who are truly handicapped. Their paralysis has become such an obstacle to them that they either withdraw from society or develop personality defects. Some see their plight as a justifiable reason to be bitter at the world and angry with God. Still others use disabilities to escape from responsibility, to avoid the daily pressures of life and work. Finally, there are those who are handicapped not by their physical disabilities but by those around them who think handicap.

I have had the experience of others attempting to impose their concept of "handicap" on my circumstances. On one occasion a well-meaning lady approached Tres just before our daughter was born. It must have taken some courage or great curiosity on her part to ask, but she said something like, "My dear, why did you and Roger decide to have a child?" It was quite obvious after several more comments that she did not feel we should have children because of what she called, my handicap. The handicap was in her mind, for our thirteen-year-old daughter, Lori, is fairly good proof of a rather normal childhood and home.

ATTITUDES AFFECT OTHERS

This same attitude can be expressed indirectly as well as directly. During the almost two years I spent in the hospital when I first had polio, one particular nurse conveyed such an understanding through her earnest desire to be helpful. Her attitude toward me was one of pity, her attempt to cater to my every need, real or anticipated, became very difficult to accept. Even her speech took on the tone of one speaking to a small child rather than to an adult.

The problem became severe enough that it began affecting my outlook and I finally had to ask the doctor to not assign her to my room. One thing a person does not need during a period of adjustment to a problem is pity. I certainly do not condemn her motive, but indirectly she was imposing the handicap of self-sympathy on me.

In my acquaintance with other physically disabled people, I know several who have self-imposed handicaps. One acquaintance refuses to get out of bed. Though this person has considerable use of arms and slight leg movement, there has been no effort to adjust to a more normal way of life. Obviously, remaining in bed day after day places far more limitations on a person than is necessary. The end product is a life of depression and a feeling of helplessness. Another acquaintance has developed such a bitter attitude about his physical problem that he has withdrawn from society altogether. It was very difficult for me to get to know this person, and required time and patience. But even when a limited amount of communication took place his bitter attitude often revealed itself.

Outside the realm of physical problems are vast areas of difficulties that would handicap each of us. In one way or another, we all are handicapped by those obstacles in life that prevent us from attaining God's perfect purpose. Is there anyone who can say, "I have achieved completely my goals in life!" or "I have done all that I can do!"? When we are honest with ourselves we cannot say that we have made our lives all that they can be. There always is room for improvement. The more practical application of life is to deal with and use these obstacles or handicaps as boosters to a more effective life. As Moses, Jeremiah, Peter, and so many more have discovered, this utilization of handicaps can be accomplished as we respond to God.

DEALING WITH HANDICAPS

In my experience of dealing with handicaps that have confronted my life, I have discovered ways of effectively dealing with and overcoming such obstacles. I do not suggest that everyone will always come out on top or achieve total victory. But as I have consciously applied these principles there has been a considerable improvement in positive results.

NEVER ALONE

First, as a Christian, I find it a significant asset to know that Jesus Christ is just as much involved in my problems as I am. At one point he said, "Come to me, all who labor and are heavy laden, and I will give you rest. . . . For my yoke is easy, and my burden is light" (Matthew 11:28, 30). What a lift it is to know that we do not face difficulties alone!

Surely we have all had a concerned friend help us solve a particular problem. On one occasion a young man in his early twenties phoned me to ask if he and his fiance could come to our home for a visit. I had not met the couple prior to this but Tres and I welcomed the opportunity to meet them. In our conversation with them we discovered that primarily they wanted to know how our marriage was working out. You see, the young man was in the same physical condition that I was. Polio had left him without much movement from his neck down. Before taking the all-important step of marriage, this young couple wanted assurance that another marriage had succeeded under similar circumstances. They eventually entered into this lifelong relationship knowing they were not alone.

We can enter into all of life's experiences knowing that Christ is with us. The handicaps we face are not insurmountable when we know we do not face them alone. The very presence of Christ lends us courage and strength to overcome.

ONE DAY AT A TIME

Not many years ago I met a middle-aged man who recently had been told he had a progressive, incurable disease. In our conversation at one point he asked, "How do you learn to cope with a physical ailment?" I had no simple answer for him, but I did suggest that facing each day as it came—my second principle—had its merits. If there is anything that will defeat us, it is to pile problem upon problem anticipating all possible complications. This makes mountains of worry out of the anthills of each day's concerns.

In Matthew 6:34 are Jesus' reassuring words,

"Therefore do not be anxious about tomorrow, for tomorrow will be anxious for itself. Let the day's own trouble be sufficient for the day." I do not feel he suggests that we should never plan ahead, but rather we should not anticipate the worries of tomorrow, today.

During my rehabilitation period I soon discovered that I had more success when dealing with one problem at a time than when looking at all of them at once. At first, all I thought about was all the things I thought I could never do again. It was an overwhelming view. It took almost three months for me to learn to "frog-breathe" (the ability to force air into my lungs by a swallowing motion). If I had known it would take that long at the beginning, I may have given up. But each day I tried it, I experienced some progress. By taking each day as it came, I realized that I could and would overcome my physical handicaps.

DEVELOP POSITIVE ATTITUDES

This brings me to the third principle: the need to develop positive attitudes. In whatever circumstance we find ourselves, it is important to dwell upon *What we can do,* not on what we cannot do! The power of positive thinking is a real force in our lives. Optimism is of optimal importance.

One of the difficulties in having a physical handicap is the tendency to be negative. For example, some will not bother to dress in a normal manner. They may be content to always wear slippers, or a robe, or not bother to take care of their hair. Some men even refuse to shave. To me it is almost like saying, "I'm handicapped and I can't help it!" Yet, I feel a positive outlook will help keep a person in as normal a circumstance as possible. Having a positive attitude includes one's appearance. I also recognize involvement as a positive attitude. Instead of confinement and limitation, the emphasis should be on go and do. The positive outlook helps us to realize how we can fit in, where we can contribute, and when we are needed.

One mother expressed herself in positive terms when she stated concerning her Mongoloid son, "The public will just have to get used to seeing my child, for I do not intend to handicap him by withdrawing him from society." It is this kind of attitude that each can apply to the handicaps we face, no matter what they are.

LEARN CONTENTMENT

Finally, I feel it is necessary to learn to be content in whatever circumstance we find ourselves. The Apostle Paul said, "Not that I complain of want; for I have learned, in whatever state I am, to be content" (Phil. 4:11). It is not that Paul was against improvement. To me he expresses that inner quality that accepts joyously the handicaps of life yet looks for the good to be accomplished.

To be content is another way of saying we are satis-fied with life. There was a time when I was not content with the results polio had thrust on my life. I fought against the very thought that I might be paralyzed the rest of my life. In the long run that fight only served to further frustrate and complicate the situation. It was not until I began to accept what would be my lot in life that I began to conquer the physical handicap.

In thinking of a handicap in terms of that which limits one from fulfilling God's full experience for each life, my physical paralysis is not a handicap. On the contrary, it is as a result of physical impairment that I have experienced a full and meaningful life with God. Though there are other obstacles that cross my path from time to time that would limit life, I cannot in all honesty say that paralysis has deprived me of a satis-fying, purposeful, happy life. What handicap is it that is a vehicle to a more complete life?

Chapter **8**

Chuckholes on Life's Road

Have you ever driven down a road full of chuck-holes? Not only must you drive the car slowly, but you must turn the steering wheel sharply to miss the deepest, most dangerous holes. There is, however, no way to miss them all. One thing as certain as death as we travel life's road is this: we will have problems!

There are two basic philosophies to adopt as we encounter each problem. We can develop a "preventive medicine" way of life, or we can just attempt to handle each difficulty as we lunge into it. The difference in these methods has to do with our general attitudes. The person holding the first view says, "By developing good mental and physical health practices I can eliminate many of life's problems." The person with the other philosophy might say, "Let's not worry about problems until we have that bridge to cross."

DEVELOP DISCIPLINES

There is much to be said for the development of personal disciplines that prevent problems we would otherwise encounter. The old saying "An ounce of prevention is worth a pound of cure" contains much truth. How much better it is to give our minds to wholesome and productive thoughts than to wade in the depths of worry or self-pity. It is far more fruitful to apply ourselves to constructive contributions to our fellowman than to approach fellowship in a critical, negative manner.

The Apostle Paul dealt with this idea when he said, "Finally, brethren, whatever is true, whatever is honorable, whatever is just, whatever is pure, whatever is lovely, whatever is gracious, if there is any excellence, if there is anything worthy of praise, think about these things. What you have learned and received and heard and seen in me, do; and the God of peace will be with you" (Phil. 4:8-9). To me Paul is saying we should avoid meditating on the unworthy aspects of life and concentrate on that which is positive and right. To practice good mental thinking is to add a quality to life that prevents many self-induced problems.

As an athlete I discovered early that a disciplined mind and body were essential to achievement. Even in college I weighed only 155 pounds (soaking wet) and stood five feet eight inches tall (in shoes). Some persons along the way had said my size would prevent me from becoming much of an athlete. But early in high school I decided to apply that extra amount of discipline that would overcome my lack of size.

NO SHORTCUTS

I can still hear a comment Dob Grow, my college football coach, made during one of his preseason chalkboard sessions. He said, "In order to play this game well, you've got to be honest!" The obvious point is that there are no shortcuts to becoming a good player. It must be done by spending hour after hour on the fundamentals of running, passing, blocking, tackling, timing, and body conditioning. Because of the philosophy I had decided upon earlier, I can truthfully say that my size was never a detriment to my sports career. The problem never existed except in the minds of a few skeptics.

Now that I am physically handicapped I can see even more clearly the importance of good mental health. During the early stages of paralysis I often had the frustration of wanting to move—just to move a hand or an arm would have satisfied me. It was difficult to always need someone to feed or dress me. The iron lung was depressing and it was easy to allow my thoughts to become bitter and resentful.

I will never cease to be amazed at the change Jesus Christ brought to my mind and life when he became my Lord and Savior. It was like lifting a shade in a darkened room to let the bright sunlight burst in. Almost instantly I began to see life from a new frame of mind. I am not suggesting that all my problems dissolved. But I realized that in order to overcome my circumstances, with the help of God, it could be done by looking at the positive, constructive aspects of life.

The best approach, I found, is to live life on the "high" side. That is, to maintain a positive, healthy outlook. Psychologists tell us we tend to become what we allow our minds to dwell upon. But, as I stated earlier, we all have problems at one time or another. How successful we are in dealing with them depends on our perspective. Do we view troubles and difficulties with disdain or do we see them as a potential for growth and maturity?

The problems the world faces today can either overwhelm and defeat us or can allow us to see God working. When we rely upon news reports, there is much to be discouraged about, for many problems seem unsolvable. Yet there is much good happening in our world as well. You and I can decide whether to be critical and condemning or to be contributors in the search for solutions to these problems.

Individual problems often are reflections of the times. But it is here—on the personal level—that we must learn to deal with our troubles.

It is apparent to me there are two basic methods to use in dealing with personal problems: (1) to find the resources within ourselves to satisfactorily solve the difficulty; (2) to seek outside sources to help deal with the problem. In either case our relationship with God has far-reaching implications. To consider running away from or setting aside a problem has no merit and will only compound the difficulty.

To illustrate these two methods, I would like to share the experience of two of our close friends. The procedure they followed fits the pattern.

This couple, prior to the time they began attending church, was having marriage problems. The problem had compounded itself to the point it was carrying them to the brink of divorce. Attempts to talk out their differences went on for months, with no apparent progress or solution in sight. As the problem became more desperate both husband and wife began to look in other directions for the answer.

During one particular disagreement, the husband turned to the Bible to lend support to his argument. Up to this point, neither partner felt any need for the church, much less a living relationship with God. What my friend found, however, was not support for his view but an insight into his own need to change. God began to work.

It was not long after this discovery that the husband decided one Sunday morning to attend church. He selected a neighborhood church only because their two children had been there on occasion. Motivated by the hope that maybe the church held the answer, he went with an open heart, seeking the solution to a worsening problem. When he returned home following the service that day and informed his wife he was going back the next Sunday, she responded with an affirmative, eager desire for them to pursue this avenue together.

The following week the four went to church as a family. It was not many weeks later that both husband and wife had given themselves to God in a commitment to Jesus Christ. It signaled the beginning of the end of their marriage problem. To this day they are happy to share their experience for they have been an active, effective part of God's church.

In solving their problem, this couple first attempted to iron out the differences between themselves. When this proved ineffective they looked elsewhere. A solution was found because they were seeking an answer through one method or the other.

RESOURCES WITHIN US

One of the television commercials seen repeatedly several years ago always ended with, "But I'd rather do it myself!" When a problem confronts us, a similar reaction usually occurs. And rightly so, for we have a well of resources from which to draw. Past experiences, education, and the ability to reason and make judgments are all at our beckoning call. To add to the depth of these resouces is the presence of God within our lives. Paul states in Ephesians 3:16: "that according to the riches of his glory he may grant you to be strengthened with might through his Spirit in the inner man."

It is much like the conversion experience. Salvation begins at the point when one recognizes his need of Jesus Christ. Repentence is the next essential step, followed by genuine acceptance of Christ as Lord. Similarly, the first step in attempting to solve a problem is to acknowledge there is one. (Too often we prefer the easier route of thinking it does not exist.) Then evaluate the problem by asking how you might have caused or may contribute to the difficulty. Once done, you then can begin to face the problem squarely, whether the problem is with another person or in a circumstance. Obviously each problem is different and multifaceted. There is no sure way to predict the outcome, but I have found this simple method effective for me. Though the results are not always those desired, it nevertheless sets in motion inner resources upon which we may draw.

God's part is indicated by a statement recorded in Romans 8:28: "We know that in everything God works for good with those who love him, who are called according to his purpose." Here is an invaluable resource available to us. It is within us to love God and by so doing we have the assurance that he is striving to accomplish good even from every difficulty we face. The confidence made available to us by this knowledge adds immeasurably to the success we have in dealing with problems.

TURNING TO OUTSIDE SOURCES

Usually, not until desperation engulfs us do we begin to consider outside help for the solution to a problem. Yet, we probably could save ourselves much trouble if we were not so hesitant about seeking the counsel of others.

As a ninth grader in high school I was faced with the problem of making a public speech. I had been elected president of the class and was expected to give a brief talk to my classmates: almost 300 students. My homeroom teacher offered her help in my preparation for the occasion, but I was at that age where I did not feel help was needed. At the ripe old age of fourteen I figured I was capable of handling the situation.

When the time arrived, I walked to the podium with fear and trembling. I had not prepared too well and I knew it. As the first few words left my mouth, my mind suddenly went blank. I quickly looked back at my teacher sitting halfway back in the auditorium as if to say, "What should I do now?" All I could see was her face slowly sinking into the palms of her hands. That speech died before it really was born.

Though this was not the most serious problem I faced, I did learn that I could profit by accepting advice from others. In Proverbs 19:20 are the words, "Listen to advice and accept instruction, that you may gain wisdom for the future."

When problems of a serious nature confront us, it

is often wise to seek counsel from someone in whom we have confidence. There are many sources to which we can turn—to friends as well as professionals. Woven throughout these periods of stress and strain is the vital need for communication with God. While we seek outside sources, God is also working to bring about the proper answers.

The life of Helen Keller is a good example of one who used both approaches to solving an almost overwhelming problem. Her faithful friend and nurse provided an outside source of help that allowed Miss Keller to "hear" and speak, though she was deaf from birth. But also there was her inner strength and courage at work contributing to the solution of the problem. At the core of her life was Helen's deep, active relationship with God.

How important it is for each of us to develop a healthy attitude toward problems. Without doubt we will have them. Success in our search for solutions will depend much upon personal insights. Each experience should be measured not only by end results but also by the question, Has it made me a better person? My personal experience is that no difficulty is insurmountable when we approach it in harmony with God and in the proper frame of mind.

Chapter **9**

Upon This I Will Build!

It has been my experience that being involved in church activity is essential to a Christian's growth. Yet, there seems to be an aversion by many members to become a part of the church's total ministry. This is plainly evident when we read such statements as "Twenty percent of the church members are responsible for eighty percent of the jobs." According to many religious leaders today, the same disparity exists in the areas of financial support and the use of special talents. Why is this and what can be done about it?

FAST-PACED LIVING

There is no doubt that the society in which we live is moving rapidly. The attractions and pull of many functions and activities from all sides are bound to take their toll on the church. One of my high school friends returned to South Bend after working in San Francisco for several years. He acknowledged that while he was enjoying his visit home, he already missed the hectic, "going every minute" life he had just left. "There is so much to do there, with lots of things going on!" he wistfully related.

The pace of life, of course, has increased in nearly all cities and towns. Where the church was often the center of social and religious activities, now it is just one of numerous activities. We who attend church and are involved must now make choices about how we will divide our time. Rightly so, for Christians need to be a part of what is going on. Our children are busier today, with many school and community activities. Politics requires our interest, if not our participation. Often we are required to spend more time at jobs and their related demands. Squeezed into what spare time is left are social obligations to relatives, friends, and neighbors. Moreover, the church asks not only for our attendance, but also our involvement.

DETERMINE PRIORITIES

The answer is found in determining priorities. We must ask, What is more important? We must search for the solution to the question, How can I best utilize my time?

In Matthew 16:17-18 Jesus said to Peter, "Blessed are you, Simon Bar-Jona! For flesh and blood has not revealed this to you, but my Father who is in heaven. And I tell you, you are Peter, and on this rock I will build my church, and the powers of death shall not prevail against it." He was saying that because of such faith as Peter's, the church would make its foundation. The church is built upon the faith that Christ is who he said he was. It is structured by the faith we have in the living God. Here is where we must begin to evaluate our church relatedness.

MY CHURCH INVOLVEMENT BEGINS

My church involvement began shortly after Tres and I came to South Bend. Reverend Larry Reynolds, then pastor of a south side church, asked one day if I was interested in typing a stencil for the Sunday church bulletin each week. At that stage I was not sure just what I could do for the church. But since I could type I felt it would at least occupy some of my idle time.

Not many months later I was asked to help teach a junior boys' Sunday school class. I accepted, but reluctantly, thinking it might be difficult to get to church so early every Sunday. (It normally requires about two hours for Tres to get both of us ready to attend church.)

Within the following year, however, I not only had taken over the teaching job, but we were attending morning and evening services on Sunday and the midweek prayer service. One thing led to another, and it was not long until I had accepted responsibilities on several committees. Over these past sixteen years,

Tres and I have been active in teaching, evangelism, church council, office chores, and coaching the softball and basketball teams. It has required much time but we consider it as part of our ministry for Jesus Christ.

I must interject at this point that we did not consistently make the proper choices with our time. There was a period when church work took so much of our time there was little left for friends or other involvements. It was not unusual for us to have five nights out of seven tied up in one way or another at church. During this time I had what seemed to be a casual enough experience, but which to this day serves as a reminder for me to keep priorities in line.

INTERFERENCE EVALUATED

A number of my high school buddies were to play in the preliminary basketball game scheduled prior to the Globe Trotters. The game was being played at one of the local schools and I had mentioned to one friend that it might be fun to see the game. A week or so later I received a phone call from one of my friends inviting me to attend. He explained that the fellows would make all the necessary arrangements and would have several guys at the door to help get me into the building. It all sounded great—until the date was mentioned. Suddenly I realized that the game would be on Wednesday night: prayer meeting night!

I quickly declined the invitation, explaining that I had to attend church that evening. I can still hear my friend's reply: "Church is a good thing, but you shouldn't overdo it!" I held to my decision, but I went to church that particular Wednesday with mixed emotions.

In recalling this incident, I cannot agree with the attitude in which my friend's statement was made, but it was made with some basis in truth. It made me begin to consider some very basic philosophies about church involvement. Perhaps the midweek service was the better choice at that time, but what about the opportunity I had bypassed to associate with non-Christians? I also realized that my involvement with those outside the church was limited, almost to the point of nil. Then it dawned upon me that the real purpose of the church is not simply to have meetings, services, and fellowship with other Christians. It is to provide the witness we bear as we go into all the world.

PROPER PERSPECTIVE

This may be where many church members get "hung up." Too often the tendency is to substitute building-oriented involvement for the task Christ asks each of us to perform. Many persons see the church as nothing more than a religious social order and refuse to become a part. Others become so involved in and bogged-down with organization-related responsibilities that they lose sight of the real purpose. Their energy is drained. Somewhere in each Christian's life is a balance. The balance depends upon our desire to be a link between God and the world and our perspective of how the church accomplishes this goal.

Paul stated the purpose of the church quite clearly in 2 Corinthians 5:18-20. "All this is from God, who through Christ reconciled us to himself and gave us the ministry of reconciliation; that is, God was in Christ reconciling the world to himself, not counting their trespasses against them, and entrusting to us the message of reconciliation. So we are ambassadors for Christ, God making his appeal through us."

If we want the church to become a meaningful part of our lives, we must build upon this foundation. We need to see the church as a collective body of individual Christians seeking to take Jesus Christ to the world, the unsaved. It is this thriving, living faith that should underscore our investment of time, talents, and money.

EACH IS NEEDED

The church needs you and me to be an active part of its total program. We need to support the many activities with our presence, but not necessarily each time the doors open. For the sake of the church and its effectiveness, we need to set priorities, remembering that we must allow time for family relationships as well as friends and neighbors. By so doing we extend the arm of the church outward beyond its walls to the appointed destination.

Pastor Edward Bruerd, formerly serving in South Bend, felt that one of his tasks was to help each Christian see his or her ministry outside as well as inside the church. It was he, for example, who initiated the idea of a church softball team that eventually led to the conversion of a family in our church.

Bill Grenert began attending our church softball games because two of his brothers played on our team. Not many weeks later, Bill expressed an interest in joining the team. We all encouraged him to come out to practice, but there was one league rule he had not met: a player must attend church services at least twice a month.

Bill readily agreed to meet that condition. He, his wife Edna, and their five children began attending church regularly. Their attendance exposed them each week to the message of salvation, and to the fellowship of believers. By the end of the year they all had given their lives to Jesus Christ. I am not suggesting that softball alone brought them to the point of conversion. But the activity was certainly instrumental in bringing about exposure to the real purpose of the church. I might add that over the thirteen years we have had a sports program in our church, we have touched the lives of more than fifty young men. Admittedly, most associations have not led to the dramatic results Bill and his family experienced, but each man was witnessed to in one way or another through fellowship and in attending church services.

PROGRAMS USED FOR GOD

If sports can be used for God, how much more can our programs of evangelism, worship, music, and missions be of value in building the Kingdom! The church needs faithful, dedicated volunteers to function within the framework of its program. But we also must recognize, *we* need the church! We each must realize that it is vital to our growth and expression as individual followers of Christ. It is here that we should build and develop the materials with which to structure our lives in the world.

Following a visit to a church in southern Indiana, I was approached by a man with tear-brimmed eyes. Placing a warm hand on my shoulder, he said, "I feel ashamed of myself after hearing all the activities you are involved with in your church."

After assuring him that that was not my purpose in sharing such information, I told him, "I do it because God has done so very much in my life!" Really, how can we who have experienced and seen God working do less than give ourselves to the ministry of the church?

As for me and my family, we will build our lives upon this!

Chapter **10**

Implementing a Generous Spirit

Generousness takes may forms. It is much like viewing a diamond with a magnifying glass. Each facet glows in a unique and distinct manner. A generous spirit reveals itself in an act of forgiveness, in willingness to overlook another's shortcomings. It is seen in an expression of giving, or an attitude of understanding. Wherever it is found you will recognize one basic truth woven throughout each pattern: it is characterized by the desire to add to the well-being of others.

Someone has said "Generosity begins at the point of sacrifice." Opportunities to give come to us in many ways. Your mailbox is probably as full as mine when it comes to requests for donations. Our churches need our faithful, consistent giving of tithes and offerings in order to fulfill their mission. Then there is the gift of talents which must be considered along with time. However or whenever we give, it is the chance to exercise a generous spirit. I discovered this in a very unusual way one Wednesday evening eight years ago.

GENEROSITY DEMONSTRATED

During the midweek service an unshaven, poorly-dressed, middle-aged man wandered into our church. Apparently not too sure of where he was and obviously under the influence of alcohol, he hesitantly made his way to a chair near me. Throughout the remainder of the service he seemed engrossed in his own problems, talking to himself and occasionally mentioning God. Periodically he would interrupt himself, lean toward me, and mumble what sounded like a prayer.

When the service ended, he again directed his attention my way. He spoke in halting phrases that sounded something like, "You'll be all right!" and "I'm praying for you!" Without much hesitation he then reached deep into his tattered and torn coat pocket, pulled out a large red apple, and handed it to me.

My first reaction was to say no, for it was obvious he had little else to eat. But, on second thought, it occurred to me that here was an expression of generosity, a sacrifice on his part. I thanked him and he placed the apple in my lap. Seemingly satisfied, he then left to make his way back out to the highway to continue his journey. I never saw him again.

To this day I recall with amazement the generous attitude of this man. In spite of the despair and adversity his life obviously portrayed, from the depths of his soul came the spark of a generous spirit. Perhaps it was not exactly the widow's mite, but it was an act of sacrifice prompted by generosity.

SEEK THE GOOD

Another facet of a generous spirit is seen in an attitude that seeks the good in every experience. It is that spirit which makes allowances for shortcomings and turns criticism into constructive happenings. I learned this invaluable attribute one Sunday morning while worshiping with friends.

Bill and Eddy Lisenko were visiting us from Chicago on this particular weekend. It happened that we were having a special musical group as the worship program, music the style of which I was not especially fond. Halfway through the service I turned to Bill and made a wry face of disapproval. I was not enjoying it but merely enduring it.

Later that same day Bill told me, "Man, you sure took me off cloud nine! I was really enjoying myself!" I suddenly realized that my spirit in that instance had not been one of generousness. Because the music had not suited my taste, I was ready and willing to detract from the musicians' efforts to serve Jesus Christ. Bill told me he felt it was a matter of making a conscious effort to gather that which is good from all experiences. From that day on I have made an attempt to enjoy and appreciate all sincere forms of worship, in spite of my personal likes and dislikes.

UNDERSTAND OTHERS

The facet of understanding one another is a daily struggle to develop. It is not so difficult when we view things from an objective perspective. But, when a situation becomes subjective to the point we are on the receiving end of an injustice, then understanding is the result of a generous spirit. It was in this vein that Tres had an experience with our daughter Lori a few years ago.

It had been raining this particular day so Tres decided to drive Lori home in the car after school. As usual, many other parents had the same idea in mind. Cars jammed the street for an entire block around the school. After fighting the traffic for fifteen minutes, Tres pulled up to the curb. But Lori was not in sight. Another fifteen minutes went by before she appeared at the school door. Happy to see her mother still there, she bounded to the waiting car.

Upon entering, however, Lori found a very unhappy mother. Tres was upset for having to wait so long. It was damp and cold and there was no apparent reason for Lori to be so late leaving school, Tres thought. They were almost home by the time she had finished her lecture punctuated by, "Why weren't you ready when I got there?" and "You should be more considerate of others!" Lori sat silently, listening, not able to get in a word of defense edgewise.

Finally noting that her mom was through, she leaned over and kissed Tres. The kiss as much as said, "Mom, I know you're irritated and I understand, but I still love you!" We later learned that Lori's tardiness had been justified. And instead of reacting in anger to the bawling-out, she implemented a generous spirit. (To be sure, our family "discussions" do not always turn out this way.)

FORGIVE GENEROUSLY

One of the brightest facets of a generous spirit is forgiveness. Jesus' emphatic words recorded in Matthew 6:14 state, "For if you forgive men their trespasses, your heavenly Father also will forgive you; but if you do not forgive men their trespasses, neither will your Father forgive your trespasses." This is not a bargain to take or leave. It is a basic principle God has set in motion, and upon which we can build relationships.

A year after we returned to South Bend from my hospital stay, an acquaintance asked to talk with us about something very important. When she, Tres, and I were alone, she began by asking us to forgive her. Apparently over a period of time some feelings of resentment had built up, though we had not been aware of it. After a time of open discussion concerning the possible cause and reasons for such feelings, the problem was resolved in an atmosphere of forgiveness. We parted having found an even stronger friendship based on an inner spirit of generosity.

SOURCE OF GENEROUSNESS

To discover the source of a generous spirit I find it helpful to turn to the fourth chapter of First John. The entire chapter has to do with our spirit and how it is an expression of God's love for us and ours for others. In particular, verses 12 and 13 declare, "No man has ever seen God; if we love one another, God abides in us and his love is perfected in us. By this we know that we abide in him and he in us, because he has given us of his own spirit."

Love is at the very heart of generosity. It is the result of God's indwelling Spirit in your life and mine. Without his Spirit we are left with a rather shallow, ineffective generousness. Our reactions to injustices and shortcomings become ill-tempered. It is easier to strike out at others in criticism, to lose patience, to condemn. But when we exert the power of love for one another that God makes available, we find a storehouse of generosity.

Some of the best examples of just such a generous spirit I've experienced over the years have come from my own friends. As a result of my physical disability, I have been in a unique position to receive many kindnesses and considerations. The thoughtfulness of most people is truly gratifying, though it is not always easy for me to be a gracious receiver. There have been a few persons along the way who attempted to exploit my circumstances, but most have at least been well-intentioned.

My friends, however, are to me a rather special breed. Our relationships, for the most part, have been on the basis of mutual interests and respect. Other than the obvious physical limitations on my part, most interrelations have been on a give-'n-take level. Of course, many friends go beyond generousness to be of help, or to add to my comfort. But the fact that I am accepted and treated as an equal—not as an invalid—has been a blessing to my life. Too often there is the tendency to pamper or pity and sympathize with a handicapped person. This is one thing that is not needed, and usually is not wanted. It is only as an individual is able to gain a degree of self-respect and self-worth that he is able to become a whole being.

I sincerely feel that my life would not be satisfying and complete without the healthy, generous spirit expressed by friends. It is that kind of spirit of love and concern that desires the best for another. Herein is the key that unlocks the diamond of many facets: generousness.

A generous spirit bridges the gap of bad feelings. It turns short tempers into patience and makes allowance for mistakes. Injustices become opportunities to deeper understanding or to experience the healing power of forgiveness. This and much more become ours as a result of God's abiding Spirit.

A generous spirit carries us through the realm of giving to sacrifice. Time, talents, and possessions are gifts to be shared. The times we desire to strike out in self-defense are turned into moments of constructive action. Interrelations with our fellowman are based upon trust and the desire for his best interest. All this and still more is ours when we implement our lives with the indwelling Spirit of God.

Chapter *11*

Play to Win!

Why does one man fail and another succeed? Why is one Christian running over with enthusiasm and another seemingly empty and dry? Obviously there are no pat answers to these questions, for there are many influences at work. The search for the victorious life, however, is one that goes on throughout a lifetime.

STRIVE FOR VICTORY

The word *victory* denotes a sense of overcoming, winning, or succeeding at an endeavor. Victory is that something we are taught to strive for from childhood. As a former athlete and current armchair quarterback, I have tasted the sweet fruits of victory as well as the bitter gall of defeat. The object in sports is to win. The hours of disciplined practice are geared to achieve victory over the opponent. As the late Vince Lombardi put it, "Winning isn't everything. It's the only thing!"

Probably the most thrilling victory I was involved in was a football game during my sophomore year in college. We traveled to Hillsdale College (Michigan), rated as one of the stronger small college teams in the Midwest that year. It was Hillsdale's homecoming and we were anticipating a difficult Saturday afternoon in front of the hometown crowd.

The first half of the game went as expected; Hillsdale was leading by a score of 21 to 7. Their huge line had made gaping holes in our defense. Offensively, we had real difficulty even moving the ball against the giant defensive line. We were being beaten and there was not much doubt in the minds of the Hillsdale fans.

During the half-time intermission our coach did not give us one of those so called pep-talks. Instead, he set out to correct our errors, and showed us where their weaknesses were. He discussed the plays we would run in the second half and adjusted our defense to stop Hillsdale's running game. When we left the dressing room to go back onto the field, we knew what had to be done to win.

The second half began. We gained possession of the ball and marched to a touchdown. The score now read: 21 to 14. But when we kicked off, Hillsdale proceeded to return the ball for another score, much to our disappointment. Their kicker, however, missed the extra point and we trailed, 27 to 14. At the beginning of the fourth period we again made a sustained drive for another touchdown pulling us within striking distance. The scoreboard revealed a 27 to 21 tally. After kicking off again our defense held Hillsdale and they had to punt. At this point Coach Grow employed a play he felt would work due to a weakness he spotted in their defense. The play not only was responsible for a seventy yard touchdown run, but for the ultimate victory. We defeated Hillsdale 28 to 27! What a thrill it was for me to be part of such a team effort. It all had been achieved because each of us had played to win!

A dedicated athlete knows he must train and prepare in order to be on a winning team. It should be the same for a Christian. To live the Christian life with sparkle and that something extra, requires much time spent in preparation. Success in business is achieved by planning and hard work. Effectiveness as one of Christ's followers is the result of efforts put forth to meet life. One of the quotes I have found most meaningful is, "What you are is God's gift to you. What you make of yourself is your gift to God!" To accomplish the desired results in life, we must play to win.

MAINTAIN OPTIMISM

Several people over the years of my paralysis have asked me, "How do you manage to maintain a happy outlook on life in spite of your handicap?" My usual reply is that I certainly do not have a corner on the market, but victorious living is available to all, under any circumstances. My conviction is that one reason for a person's lack of victory in life is his not knowing how to face and overcome tribulations. Without problems there is the tendency to coast along taking all good fortunes as they come. But when confronted by troubles, the failure to have prepared for such times defeats us.

Jesus Christ made a sort of summarizing statement to his disciples in John 16:33 when he said, "I have said this to you, that in me you may have peace. In the world you have tribulation; but be of good cheer, I have overcome the world." The apparent emphasis was on overcoming life's trials and difficulties.

In my attempts to evaluate and determine how to live life on the plus side, I have made several personal discoveries. I would like to share these findings with you in this final chapter.

TROUBLES STRENGTHEN

In an earlier chapter I wrote about the importance of dealing with problems. It has been my experience to find difficulties a real source of strength for all of life. They can be a step up to a more meaningful existence.

Several years ago I re-met a friend with whom I had attended elementary and high school. We talked at length about old times and the present. When our visit ended he said, "Man, you sure have changed!"

More recently I met another ex-schoolmate following a church service in which I had spoken. Her comment was, "You're a lot different from when I knew you before!" Their apparent reference was to the difference in attitudes and philosophy I had now as compared to my life before polio.

In all honesty I can say that my physical affliction has made me a better, happier person. At the time it occurred I felt my disability was the worst that could possibly happen. But in those days of desperate searching for the answer to the riddle, "Why me," I turned to God. It is likely that I would not have changed my basic outlook on life if it had not been for this illness. Forced by necessity to face the problem, I found a source of inner strength previously unknown to me.

Tribulations often can be the stimulators that trigger action. When we have a problem to work against, it stimulates us to seek a solution. Just as an antagonistic muscle is essential to the effective movement of a primary muscle, so trials serve to help us flex to meet life as it comes. William Barclay says it this way, "The Christian is the athlete of God whose spiritual muscles become stronger from the discipline of difficulties."

Tres and I had occasion to meet a charming young lady who had been selected as the Goodwill Worker of the Year in 1965. Karla Hambel, then twenty-three years old, was born without arms, but her hands are attached at the shoulders. In addition, one leg is deformed and three inches shorter than the other. Considering the handicap, logic almost dictates that Karla would be destined to an abnormal, maladjusted life.

Labeling herself "stubborn," Karla determined at an early age that nothing would stop her from becoming a productive, independent person. In time she learned to feed herself, and to walk with the aid of braces. These accomplishments allowed her to begin public school by the time she was in the eighth grade. Upon graduating as salutatorian she went on to Otterbein College (Ohio) where in four years she earned a degree in education. Because of what some termed her unacceptable physical condition, Karla was unable to find employment in the field for which she had trained. It was at this point that she turned to Goodwill Industries. She was hired immediately to do clerical work, but she soon developed an interest in counseling handicapped individuals. This then led her to enter Kent State University to do graduate study in rehabilitative counseling.

I do not believe there is any doubt that Karla Hambel found strength from her handicap. It is also apparent that her relationship to and faith in God are integral parts of the force motivating her to achievement. She has risen above her problem and has become a positive influence in our society.

DON'T FEAR TROUBLE

Though troubles are not something we seek, there is no reason to fear them. For in facing and learning to overcome problems, we discover insights into how to live day by day, satisfyingly and joyously. The strength generated from such experiences becomes preparation essential for us to live victoriously under any and all circumstances.

The Apostle Paul dealt with many difficulties throughout his lifetime. He was beaten on numerous occasions, stoned, shipwrecked, in danger at sea and from robbers, ridiculed, imprisoned. Through it all he was able to say, "More than that, we rejoice in our sufferings, knowing that suffering produces endurance, and endurance produces character, and character produces hope, and hope does not disappoint us, because God's love has been poured into our hearts through the Holy Spirit which has been given to us" (Romans 5:3-5).

COMMIT YOURSELF

There seems to be a fad today to take up a cause—any cause—and then to march on behalf of it. To commit yourself is in itself a healthy thing. But to give yourself to just any purpose that comes along is like the story I heard about a young man sitting in front of a college administration building. The forlorn-looking youth was holding a blank placard. When finally he was asked why it was blank, he mumbled, "Oh, I'm just waiting for the next cause to come along!" Fortunately, most youths are too intelligent to be led into that kind of trap.

Peter Marshall once offered the prayer, "Lord, give us courage to stand for something, lest we fall for anything." How often have you seen people blown about from one idea or philosophy to another because they lacked convictions? Without convictions we are likely to either avoid commitment or to follow the first cause that crosses our path.

To live victoriously, I find it necessary to be committed, to give myself in various ways to causes which benefit our fellowman. For me personally, the church provides the greatest service opportunities, through its many avenues of outreach. Fundamentally, the church strives to bring the message of salvation to all men as well as meet physical needs. But certainly this is not the only significant manner in which to be committed to purposeful causes.

One of the minor frustrations I encounter is to meet persons who have the impression that, because I cannot move my arms, and must use a respirator, I spend most of my time watching television or sleeping. The fact of the matter is, that kind of life would be completely unacceptable to me. I have found that being busy, involved, is a source of happiness. Idleness leads to depression and meaninglessness, but giving time and effort to my work, church, community causes, and to the welfare of friends and neighbors, produces a life well spent. This kind of life makes me eager to greet each day with renewed vigor and enthusiasm.

Paul made an appeal to the Christians in Rome to commit their lives to real purpose: He wrote, "I appeal to you therefore, brethren, by the mercies of God, to present your bodies a living sacrifice, holy and acceptable to God, which is your spiritual worship" (Romans 12:1). Paul was suggesting strongly that Christians need to give their lives to the ultimate cause of serving God. Even to the extent that it might bring physical death. He knew the perils they faced. He also knew that, for them to have victory in life, they would have to commit themselves entirely to God, even to the extent of sacrifice.

I am not suggesting that you or I should rush into needless activity every hour of every day. Yet, from personal experience it is evident to me that we need to give ourselves to worthy and constructive activities. The victorious life is one that discovers ways of being a contributor to the welfare of those around it. Until we are thus committed we will lack the ingredient that adds the spark to a winning outlook on life.

History portrays men and women who gave themselves to causes, both good and bad. The early period of our country's history records many who believed strongly in the basic freedoms upon which our nation was founded. Perhaps Nathan Hale best exemplified the commitment of those early leaders when he said, "I only regret that I have but one life to lose for my country!" As Christians we have an even greater reason and cause to which to commit ourselves. Serving God and being an asset to our fellowman and our environment go hand in hand.

CHRIST THE VICTOR

Finally, we must have a living relationship with Jesus Christ to achieve a victorious life. Not a relationship based on family ties, or custom, or convenience, but one formed as a result of intimate, personal encounter with him. This is a spiritual law that God has established which works with as much certainty as nature's law of gravity.

Jesus' remark in John 16:33 is the basis upon which you and I can claim victory within our lives. The Amplified Bible states it this way, "In the world you have tribulation and trials and distress and frustration; but be of good cheer—take courage, be confident, certain, undaunted—for I have overcome the world—I have deprived it of power to harm, have conquered it [for you.]" Jesus prepared for the battle and eventual triumph as he prayed and ministered during his earthly walk. We now have this foundation to build upon. Following Christ's example, we, too, can play to win.

I once received a letter, part of which read, "God can't use you until you are healed!" I have thought back to that statement many times, reflecting on all that has happened in my life since that day. It is obvious now that the author of the letter had underestimated God. When conditions are set by man, they limit the power of Christ within us. Until we recognize that God will use all who are willing to be used, we miss the mark of what Jesus accomplished. And what he enables us to accomplish.

I can truthfully say that I have overcome the stigma of being completely paralyzed. Though I cannot lift a finger or breathe without conscious effort or mechanical aid, I am content in knowing there is much more to life. In each chapter of this book I have shared experiences and philosophies based upon which I find life victorious. Each chapter-theme—attitudes, freedoms, witnessing, God's will, healing by grace, problems, church involvement, generousness—is integrated into my relationships with God and with my fellowman. It is here that I now "play to win"!

One of the most significant aspects I've discovered about the Christian life is to know that Jesus makes it possible for us to live in fullness and completeness wherever we find ourselves. No situation is insurmountable, for God has made a way. No life is worthless, for he establishes its value. Though we cannot continually travel on mountaintops, each problem, each challenge, each experience can help prepare us to reach new heights. Victory comes when we have learned to trust day by day what God reveals to us.

What Jesus Christ has done in my life is to convert a potential tragedy into a meaningful, joyful event.

Though I cannot foresee what is in the future for me, I can say with conviction that I would not change the past. I look forward with greater anticipation than ever to the life ahead. I yearn for new insights, new struggles, and new victories. It matters not that I may not walk today, for with Christ I'll walk tomorrow!